The Art of Microblading

Secrets from the Founder of World Microblading For Everyone From Beginner to Pro

By Irina Wynn

This book is dedicated to a man who doesn't need my praise or my exaltation. He was the very first person to believe in me—even when I had nothing but a dream. When even my own mother thought I was chasing a fool's errand, he saw the sparkle in my eyes and stuck around for the fireworks.

It's through the pages of this book that I want to thank my dear friend Manuel J., the man whose unending support inspired me to believe that I was capable of building what I have created to this day.

The Art of Microblading

Secrets from the Founder of World Microblading For Everyone From Beginner to Pro

By Irina Wynn

Table of Contents

THE ART OF MICROBLADING

Introduction
What's Your Superpower?

This Is Where We Begin...

My story is an intriguing one, full of twists and turns, of sadness and betrayal...but most of all, of triumph. If the past decade of my life has taught me anything, it is that determination is, without a doubt, a person's most important asset.

"Whether you think you can, or you think you can't...you're right."

-Henry Ford

To me, this quote screams volumes. When you put your mind to something, you have to **really** put your mind to it. You can't do it halfway and expect amazing results. You can't just give a small bit of effort and ask for a mountain of success. You have to go all in. You have to put your heart, your mind, your sweat, and your tears into something in order to see a positive outcome.

And most importantly of all, you have to believe in yourself. If you don't believe you can do it, you have doomed your mission right from the very start.

* * *

I was blessed with an amazing ambition to succeed in life; to stop at nothing to drive myself forward toward my achievements. But guess what? You have it, too. We can all be successful if we shift the focus away from ourselves to helping others instead, and shine the spotlight on giving more than we get. Our decisions shape our future; we are always just one step away from substantial change, so use your time wisely. After all, it's your most valuable resource.

The number one question I'm asked in life is this: *How the hell have you made it so far, and with so many obstacles along the way?* I'll tell you the secret...there is no secret. You've got to simply let go of negativity, forgive those who have wronged you, but never forget the lessons you've picked up along the way. Once you've learned from mistakes, the next step is to move on. At the end of the day, you only live once—so think twice about whether you want to live a life of hatred and revenge, or simply walk away from trouble with a smile. You can't change hardships, and you certainly can't stop them from happening to you—but you can use them to your advantage. You can use negativity as fuel to propel you forward in life, but *never, ever* let it hold you back. I learned something from every trial and tribulation, carving out my character a little bit more, until finally, the finished product emerged: the woman I am today.

By choosing to learn microblading and become to best in the game at it, I changed my life drastically. Guess what? I'm actually a lawyer. But here's the hard truth: I never even picked up my law degree. Yes, the law degree I spent five years of my life working to achieve, the degree I flew back and forth to my home country of Romania to obtain, the law degree I studied long and hard to get. It's just a piece of paper somewhere that I don't even have, and that I don't even use!

Let's be honest for a moment: it takes three or four years to complete a training program in a university, depending on where in the world you're studying. Unless you're graduating from one of the top 10 universities in the world, the program you began might not be as worthwhile once you finish. We've reached a point in time when our job market is changing faster than our education programs can keep up, and unless you are constantly educating yourself, your job chances may seem slimmer and slimmer as time goes on.

This is where it's important to think about the big picture: you need to ask yourself what YOU can do, regardless of anything else, to make your mark in this world. What is your one skill, the thing you can do better than anyone else you know? Capture that energy and use it to drive you forward. Find your art and use it to your advantage.

You can go through life being an accountant, a general manager, a car salesperson, you name it—and you can make a decent living. I could have made a nice paycheck as a prosecutor with my law degree, but I would have needed to either live in Romania or start over with my education...only to make decent money. But here's the thing: I'm not interested in my life just being *decent.* I want my life to be more amazing than I could have ever dreamed.

Before you jump into a huge decision that will determine the rest of your life's path, take a moment to consider all options. Look inside yourself and really think about what you want out of life. Don't rush into a university program (especially one that will cost you tens of thousands of dollars) just because it's what you're "supposed" to do.

What's Your Superpower?

For me, it was that I learned microblading. Despite the fact that I barely perform any procedures anymore (because at this point, I'm running a multimillion dollar company), I know that no one can take that skill away from me. I may have started out making blobs that looked like sausages, but I am an artist, and one of the most respected and well-known microblading artists in the world.

This, in essence, is MY superpower, my talent, my skill set and my security. Microblading has given me not only the lifestyle that my daughter and I lead, but the security in knowing that no matter life plops onto my plate in the future, I'll be okay. Regardless of where in the world I live, microblading will always be a high-cost procedure and will always net me a generous income.

If you already have your superpower mapped out, high five for that. Go eat an ice cream, baby, you earned it. If not, don't sweat it—it's not too late to get everything figured out and gain your own lifetime security. Follow your heart, your passion, and your dreams—there's a code inside of you that only you can crack.

It's okay to fail, and it's okay to fail again, but what's not okay—unacceptable, even—is to quit. We do not quit here. We try again, and again, and *again*, until we make it. There are no limits...apart from your own beliefs. Do not limit your opportunities, and shoot for the moon. If you don't reach it, that's fine—at least you'll land among the stars.

Chapter 1
A Cut Above The Rest

Why Did I Write This Book?

I've taught microblading to artists all over the world, and one thing I learned was that so many of the students I taught lacked the business mindset to go out and build their brand.

Sure, they were talented, but talent can only get you so far in today's job market. When you're working for yourself, you need to have a double-edged sword. You need talent *and* the skill to promote yourself...otherwise, no one will know who you are!

Trust me. I've personally trained artists who had the skill and finesse to become superstars—artists with incredible techniques who could draw the thinnest, most natural-looking strokes—but never quite made it to the top. Why is that? Because they didn't know how to promote themselves. They didn't put the right amount of energy in the right places, and as a result, no one ever heard of their incredible talents.

This book is for everyone making a career of microblading, whether you're just starting out or you've been in the game for a little while and you want to change your strategies to see more success come your way. This book is your crash course on business and marketing so that you can go out into the world not only prepared to set up shop as an aesthetician, but to truly be a cut above.

If you've got this book in your hands, you're already on the right track. If I had a mentor back when I was first starting out in my career, I would have saved not only millions of dollars, but years of my life! You see, I had to figure everything out for myself, which ended up costing me *big time*…in my energy, my money, my frustration, and the most valuable resource of all (the only thing you can't get back)—my time.

So take it from me: learning how to market yourself —the right way, from the very start—is going to pay off for you and your business in the long term. Think of the big picture. How do you want your life to look in five years, ten years, fifteen years, or twenty years? What goals do you have for yourself, and for your family? Think about today, but remember that the clock runs out at midnight. The rest of your life is much more important.

Think of the Future You, and never stop until you become that sparkling version of who you want to be.

* * *

If there's one thing that will always be around, it's the beauty industry. Women will always pay top dollar for services that will make them feel beautiful, confident, and on top of the world...so why not be a part of it?

Permanent makeup adds a new level to the beauty industry. With more and more women seeking permanent makeup procedures, there are countless opportunities to grow your business and rake in revenue for yourself. When done the right way, permanent makeup is a highly lucrative field, even for someone with no prior experience.

But what does it mean to do it *right?* It means much more than just performing the procedures the correct way. You hear me: it means setting up your business with a strong foundation so that it absolutely cannot collapse. At the time of this book's writing, permanent makeup is the top-grossing service in the entire beauty industry, and I'm confident that it's not going to go anywhere for a long while. Women will always want to feel beautiful, and will always shell out the cash for it.

If you've got a business mindset and you want to make it into the big leagues, stick with me. I can promise you that by the end of this book, you'll have the blueprint to build your business from the ground up: the plan to create a rock-solid base for your future achievements.

When you bought this book, you were smart enough to realize that you can't learn microblading from the pages of a book. Just as the title of this book suggests, microblading is an art; it's a skill that takes time and practice to master. Rule number one that you'll learn during your time as a microblading artist, a business woman, and a marketing guru: **never cut corners**. Invest in proper education, work your ass off, and improve your technique. Do it right, or don't do it at all.

Can someone make millions from microblading? For sure. Been there, done that! Can you do it too? Of course you can! How? Well, keep reading…

Chapter 2
Are You All In?

Introduction to World Microblading

There has been a huge uplift in client interest for microblading service over the past few years, due to mainly to the large amounts of money I have personally invested to promote the benefits of this procedure.

Feather Eyebrows, Soft Shading, Strokes and Ombré Effect—you name it!—at the end of the day, every client wants the same thing: beautiful eyebrows. And the common link between each and every client is that they are all willing to pay their hard-earned money in order to make sure their eyebrows are taken care of beautifully.

According to the *Journal of the American Medical Association*, 65% of women admit to plucking or waxing their eyebrows. Now, let's do the math here: how many of them regret it after the fact? I'd hazard to guess that at the very least, 60% of them have screwed up their brows in some way. And here's a fact that you might know, but you might not: once you pluck your eyebrows, it's a toss-up as to whether or not they'll grow back (but it's highly possible that they *won't* grow back)!

Already, you can see why microblading is a safer choice for natural, full, beautiful-looking brows. When performed the right way, a microblading procedure lasts anywhere from 6 months to 2 years—depending on certain factors like skin type, age, and ethnicity. In addition, certain other variables like aftercare can seriously affect the staying power of the pigment in the skin, but let's not ignore the facts: microblading is, overall, much more lasting than other methods of eyebrow maintenance.

LESSON ONE: GO ALL IN

I've said it before and I'll say it again (because it really is that important): if you want to make it to the top, **you have to go all in.** And I don't mean that you need to just get a quality education in microblading by a reputable trainer. That's a start, but it's nowhere near the finish line.

When I say "all in," I mean that you're going to have to invest your time, your desire, your effort, your dedication, and your commitment to becoming an expert in your field. At the end of the day, that's all that matters: you climbing your own ladder of success is all that should concern you.

I'll be honest, outside of the permanent beauty industry, I don't think I've ever seen such a lucrative opportunity for such a low price to become certified. Here's what I mean: as an aesthetician, you make more than a trial lawyer per hour, and it only costs a few thousand bucks to get certified. Ready for the cherry on top? The certification process takes five days (instead of a few years), and you don't even have to pass the bar exam! Pretty sweet deal, right?

And yet, some of you still might be saying to yourselves that a university degree is the way to go. Take it from me—the woman who spent five years traveling across Europe to go to school to obtain a law degree—I say hell no. It's not worth it, not by a long shot.

Like I said in the introduction to this book, I'm a lawyer by trade…but I never even picked up my diploma once I earned it. Why? Because by the time I was finished with my studies, I was already an entrepreneur, owning and operating salons in Norway. That's right: a Romanian lawyer was running beauty studios in Norway with ZERO previous experience, learning permanent makeup techniques on the side. What use did I have for my law degree at that point? I'll tell you: none.

This is my point: unless you graduate at the top of your class from a prestigious university, you're probably going to get lost in the shuffle of all the other graduates out there. Skills tend to fade, and even geniuses go unnoticed in such a rapidly-changing world.

This is why I say that education never stops. You have to always be on the lookout for new ways to expand your mind, and you have to always, always, *always* want to learn. It's the only way to make it in the business world.

When I announced that I was switching gears, no one believed in me, not even my own mother. I still remember her words to me:

You are becoming an aesthetician instead of a judge? Are you out of your mind?!

Those around me began to throw bricks at me, truly believing that I was making the biggest mistake of my life. But guess what? I picked up every single brick they threw my way and used them to build one of the largest vocational schools that teaches microblading (and one of the only legitimate ones, at that) in the United States of America.

What I taught was, initially, a trend—but before long, this "trend" became so popular that it was requested by Hollywood celebrities as one of the most wanted beauty services. This surge in popularity created millions of dollars in revenue for our former students and put microblading on the map as a service that won't be going anywhere anytime soon. It's for this reason that I never trust that a trend will remain temporary—my business is living proof that fads don't always fade.

If you need another example, just take a look at Bitcoin. You don't need me to illustrate how powerful cryptocurrency is—its power speaks for itself. I mean, it's digital and nonexistent, and yet Bitcoin has become one of the strongest threats to the financial industry despite all the regulations, rumors, and attempts to bash it. The same analogy holds true for microblading. As much as outsiders try to knock microblading down, its demand only increases.

Chapter 3
If The Rules Don't Work For You, Then Change The Game

How Did This Happen (And Why Did I Choose Microblading As A Career)?

You know how most awesome things in life seem to pop up from a really shitty experience? This is how I got my start as a Permanent Makeup Artist: after throwing 600 Euros down the drain. It was, quite possibly, the worst way to spend €600, but at the same time, it was the best motivation for me to succeed and prove to everyone— even myself—that I can make it in this industry.

Long story short, here's what I was taught in this "permanent makeup master course": I learned nothing but how to cross pathogens, contaminate the area, work without gloves, forgo basically *any* type of decent protection, and how to mutilate someone's face.

Oh, and as an added bonus, this instructor gave all her students a lesson in gossip with a concentration on making them feel like idiots. I left that class feeling like a loser who would never be able to tattoo anyone's eyebrows. Pretty cool deal, right?

Here's something to remember: if any "artist" ever dares to tell a novice that a person is born with a talent to perform microblading—and you either have the talent or you don't—that's bullshit. Remember my words: that's the most ridiculous thing you can hear in the entire beauty industry; it's just someone else's insecurity coming out to make you feel low and make you give up.

The sad truth is that some artists will, actually, sink that low. And yes, some artists are indeed quite talented, but it doesn't mean that someone else can't reach that same level with a whole lot practice and just as much patience. Case in point: when I first began my journey in permanent makeup, my hands were so unsteady that I created blobs that looked like sausages! And forget clean, crisp strokes—I couldn't even draw a Christmas tree!

The good news is that microblading is a *skill*, not a talent. Just like any discipline, it is a logic pattern that, when followed correctly and practiced over time, is perfected. When you pour yourself into mastering the technique, you cannot fail.

If you've got this book in your hands, you're smart enough by now to realize that I have a zero tolerance policy when it comes to discouraging anyone's career in microblading. This career path is accessible to everyone, and so is the revenue stream that comes with it. When you have the right guidance, education, and attitude, the world is yours.

After my three-day, €600 course in microblading where I learned nothing (with the exception of what *not* to do), I left the instructor with these words: "In a few months, I will be better than you."

And sure enough, a few months later, I was considered a Master Trainer of Microblading—one of only a handful worldwide—because of work I had posted through permanent makeup forums. I didn't even have a website! This instructor grew her business by ripping off her clients; she barely taught anything in her courses, except that microblading was a talent that you are either born to do or one you'll never be able to perform.

And yes, I'll admit…I still can't draw a Christmas tree. But you know what I CAN draw? Some of the most natural-looking and beautiful brows in the world. I wasn't born with this talent; I hustled day in and day out to perfect it. I sat for hours with every kind of material I could find: chicken wings, cow leather, grapes, plastic, orange peels—you name it, I practiced my microblading technique on it. I worked 20 hours a day for years to improve my skills, all in the effort to make it to the top.

And the rest is history. I worked my ass off to crack the code on skill, and I hustled so hard that I beat the natural talent.

In short, I could have chosen not to follow my dreams, instead taking a career path in law. I could have been a prosecutor—or even a judge—but I'll be honest with you: I didn't have the patience for that. I wanted to be wealthy, and I wanted it fast. I knew the only way to get the lifestyle I wanted was to get in on the eyebrow game and do it immediately—so I went for it. Once I saw that opportunity, I couldn't ignore it. Permanent makeup is a multi-million dollar industry, and I wanted to be a part of it. Once I got my foot in the door as an aesthetician, I was unstoppable. I was all in, baby.

Chapter 4
Rome Wasn't Built In A Day

Getting My Start As A Cosmetic Tattooist

The instructor who taught me nothing but how *not* to become a permanent makeup artist (and how to rip people off for €600) used a tattoo machine to get the job done—something that I never could master.

I'll admit it, I spent hours and hours—adding up to weeks and months of my life—driving myself insane trying to practice on any sort of material I could find, and I failed every time. The vibration drove me crazy, I couldn't hold my hand still enough to draw a simple dog or a cat, let alone a natural-looking eyebrow! The more I practiced with the tattoo machine, the more frustrated and confused I became; I was sucked into this hole of spending all my energy on a method that wasn't working for me.

There's a Chinese proverb that helped guide me during this time in my life:

Draw 10,000 eggs, and after that, you will be able to draw anything.

By this point in the book, you probably know what I'm going to say next. As I mentioned in the last chapter, microblading is a skill, one that requires constant practice day in and day out. Once you devote your energy and effort to it, it will reward you with mastery. Trust me on this, because I am living proof.

For me, the "eggs" in this analogy were eyebrows. I drew at least 10,000 just to stabilize my hand, just to learn the proper way to hold the tool! And then, guess what? I realized after a while that the jerky, vibrating tattoo gun—the industry standard at the time—wasn't working for me. I wasn't successful because the tools I was using were wrong for my hands—*not* because I wasn't trying hard enough.

I set out to change the game, and revolutionize the industry standard. It didn't make sense to me that a tattoo gun was the only way to tattoo eyebrows. I reasoned that if I could draw strokes with a needle by hand—without any vibration from a machine—I could be successful. So naturally, I made that my goal.

For years, at every spare moment—day or night—you could find me practicing my strokes. I ordered thousands of custom prototype needles from all over the globe to test, and I realized the same thing—they were all poor quality. And when I say poor quality, I mean it: these tools were unsterilized, packed in bulk, no lot or manufacture dates, not even an expiration date! Basically, these needles would be laughed out of any decent health department inspection.

It was clear to me then why microblading wasn't getting off the ground: no one was making the move to take the industry to the next level. And what was so pathetic was that it would be so easy! A company just needed to professionalize a line of pro products and legitimize the trade. That was it! And yet, businesses worldwide were trying to cut corners with shoddy tools and dull, unsafe blades.

I realized that if no one else was going to invest in this incredible opportunity, it might as well be me. Almost immediately, I poured my money into developing new needles and tools that I could use to transform the way microblading was performed across the globe. I worked all day in my salons, then I'd go straight home, take care of my daughter, put her to bed, and head down to what looked more like a needle laboratory: a room downstairs full of different needle prototypes I had ordered from several hundreds of companies. That was my lounge, the place where I spent all my nights, my weekends, and every extra moment of time I had. If I wasn't at one of my beauty studios or taking care of my kid, I was down there, testing out blades.

I told you before that I used to practice strokes on all kinds of materials: leather, chicken wings, fruit… whatever I could find. But here's the sad truth: nothing works quite like human skin. You can draw 10,000 eggs on a chicken wing, but until you make that first stroke on actual human skin, you're just in practice mode.

I knew I needed to get experience under my belt. I took a deep breath and began experimenting on myself. Yes, you read that right: I used the needles I designed to cut my own skin. How could I ask my clients to trust me with their faces if I couldn't put my needles to the test on myself?

Once I developed the winning needle, I introduced microblading service to my beauty studios in Oslo…for dirt cheap. Yeah, I'm a millionaire now, but back then, I was charging 999 Norwegian crowns (equivalent to $150!) for microblading service.

This may seem like a ridiculous business strategy, but hear me out. Not only did I gain valuable experience working with clients, but I was able to double my price as I got better and better at my craft. By the time I microbladed over 20,000 eyebrows, my "slowly but surely" mindset had more than paid off.

I know what you're thinking: that's an insane price for microblading. How did I pay my bills? Why did I stoop so low? Wasn't it a waste of my time? The answer to that last question: hell no!

Yeah, I was offering microblading—one of the most expensive procedures in a beauty studio—for the price of a manicure or a massage. Why? Because I had the big picture in mind. I needed practice, I needed to master my skill, and I needed to understand how my tools worked on human skin. Not only that, but I needed to examine the healing process—let's face it, a chicken wing won't bubble up and scab!

And at the same time, I was building a treasured relationship with my clients. This is what is going to be your moneymaker. In the beauty industry, this is what keeps your clients coming back to you.

My clients understood that microblading was costly, and instead of ripping them off, I was real with them. I was genuine. I wasn't trying to squeeze money out of them or exploit them. And for that, they were grateful. They wanted to help me learn just as much as I wanted to give them beautiful eyebrows.

There's A First Time For Everything

The first client I ever microbladed walked into my studio on a Saturday morning, clearly hungover with breath that smelled far from lavender. Her eyes kept welling up with tears of pain, and her skin kept bleeding all over the workspace...but she didn't say one mean word. She was a sweetheart through the entire procedure, never complaining once.

Here's a quick tip: you can never, *ever* perform microblading on a person who has consumed alcohol or other contaminations in the previous 48 hours. First and foremost, it's dangerous for the client. Secondly, it leads to a botched microblading job!

Want to see what I mean? Just take a look at the photo of my first-ever microblading job. It speaks for itself.

37

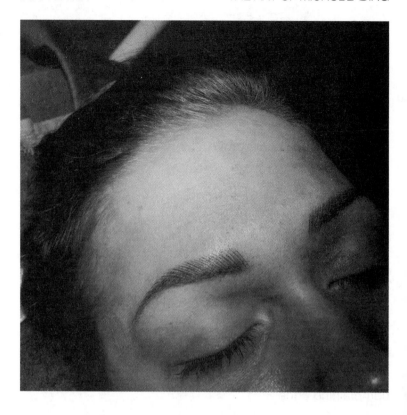

I microbladed this chick about five different times until I got her eyebrows right. And every single time, she returned to my shop with a smile—totally okay with the fact that I kept screwing up. Any other customer would storm out, pissed, and report me immediately to anyone and everyone who would listen. Not this woman; she was always humble and smiling.

In fact, when I moved from Norway to the United States, she looked at me with tears in her eyes and asked who would do her eyebrows if I moved away. Her name was Jessica, she worked as a daycare teacher, and it's truly an understatement to say that she became one of my best clients. This is what I mean about building a relationship with your customers: even though, in my eyes, I felt like I ruined this woman's eyebrows at one point, she was genuinely upset that I was leaving years later. And here I am—half a world away—and I can still vividly remember her name and her job.

You want your customers to choose *you* time after time, despite the competition. Even if the salon next to yours offers half-price microblading, or the shop down the street is giving away a free touch-up, you want to make sure that your clients are coming back to you because *they want you.*

At the end of the day, this is more than just a service performed for money. Your clients are trusting you with their faces—their windows to the world. You have an incredible power in your hands: the power to make women feel beautiful, confident, and fired up. If you can use that power wisely, you can stack your earnings higher than you dreamed, because guess what? Word of mouth is a powerful thing. If a woman is happy with the way she looks, she *will* tell her friends about it, and referrals are basically free ads with zero work! But we'll talk about that in the chapters ahead.

Here's the bottom line: bring value to peoples' lives, and you never have to worry about money for the rest of your life. You're all set, babe.

Chapter 5
Saving Eyebrows, One At A Time

Reeling In The Clients

My microblading career was on fire as soon as it began—I was booking clients 12 to 15 hours straight per day in my beauty studios! Keep in mind that I was still charging ridiculously low rates for microblading services at this time; a fraction of what someone would normally pay to get their eyebrows done professionally. What I wasn't gaining in finances, I was gaining in something far more valuable: experience.

And yeah, the main reason my schedule was so tightly packed was because I was a perfectionist who took her sweet time. Here's what I mean: if a microblading expert needed only 20 minutes to draw the perfect eyebrow set, I needed two hours. I realized that anyone can draw perfect eyebrows—whether you're a novice or a pro—by following measurements and bone features.

And after several years—don't judge, excellent things take time!—of learning, of developing my craft, I put together my own pro kit...and the shaping game was never the same. An eyebrow set that used to take me two hours had been magically cut down to ten minutes, saving me valuable time.

I had microbladed half of the faces of Oslo by the time my first few clients came back for their touch-ups four weeks after I began offering the service in my salon, and guess what? I couldn't believe how rapidly I had improved in just a few weeks! When I first began microblading, the "strokes" I made looked more like my original sausage blobs than crisp, hair-like cuts in the skin.

And yet, my customers were still so happy with the way they looked, they still smiled from ear to ear, hugged me tightly, brought me flowers, even tipped me! In Norwegian culture, this is incredibly uncommon—tipping just isn't a part of their regular routine. So naturally, if someone offered me a $50 tip at the end of a microblading service, that customer stuck out in my mind. I'd still think about that for six months, and even remember her when she came in two years later for a touch-up. A generous gift like that isn't easily forgotten.

My scrubs became my uniform—I was spending every day saving eyebrows, one at a time. I was in my early twenties at this point, and at a time in life when the women around me were still partying and getting wild on nights and weekends. I, however, had no life. Not only was I working my ass off to run my businesses and get my career as a permanent makeup artist off the ground, but I was a wife and mother. If I have to be totally honest with you, I'm not proud of some of the sacrifices I had to make in order to gain my level of success. Namely, I had to give up the opportunity to spend valuable time in the first few years of my daughter's life with her—time that she and I will never get back. But all of that is another story for another book.

One thing that I can tell you is that for all the regrets I had about rising to the top, I'm proud of what I was able to achieve. Because of my hard work and dedication, I was able to prosper and triumph in very little time, which means that these days, my daughter and I can live the life I always dreamed for us to have.

Here's the thing: I don't recommend that you take the same path I took. I had to figure things out the hard way, totally alone, and wasted millions of dollars in the process. I had no one to mentor me, no one to guide me, no one to point me in the right direction. In the long run, I ended up paying such a high price (in terms of time, energy, and money) to get to where I am today. If I had this book back then to tell me how to work smarter, not harder, it boggles my mind how much I could have saved.

So take it from me: shortcuts aren't the way to get to the top. Cutting corners and half-assing a job will only cost you more in the long run. Invest in the top quality education, tools, and supplies for your business. As I said before: do it right, or don't do it at all.

* * *

Want to know something inspiring? On average, over 80% of the work that I supervise from first-time microblading students in my training courses look far better than my first attempts back in Oslo. There's no comparison. The technique that I developed and the tools in my pro kit make it simple for anyone—even a novice—to follow the logic pattern of microblading skill and sculpt natural-looking eyebrows, even from their first try.

In fact, I was so confident in my methods that by the time I became a trainer, I offered a 100% satisfaction guarantee with every microblading course—something I still offer to this day. If any student feels as though they didn't get adequate training, we offer the course for free. To me, it was most important to blow the myth that microblading was some exclusive club you could only join if you were born with a special talent. Not in my world, baby. In my world, hard work and dedication can get you anywhere you want to go.

Chapter 6
The No-Downside Deal

Going For Groupon: Yes or No?

So, if I began with only one microblading client… you're probably wondering how my salon became overbooked with clients in just a few weeks, right? Well, here's where one of the most controversial subjects in the beauty industry comes up: Groupon. Should you do it?

I say hell yeah! Although maybe I'm a little bit biased, because that's exactly what I did. Again, my focus wasn't to earn millions at this stage, just enough to pay my bills, cover my expenses, and make sure my daughter was taken care of. I had a professional chiller husband at the time who couldn't be bothered to get a job of his own, so "bringing home the bacon," so to speak, fell on my shoulders…but that's for another book. I could write a separate book entirely about my personal story (and maybe I will one day; who knows).

This is the truth: there is no faster way to bring in more customers in bulk than Groupon. I'd use that service again and again and again, to be honest. There's virtually no downside: you have customers showing up to your door, you're getting your practice hours in, and on top of that, you're getting paid to practice! Yeah, the customers are paying a lower rate, but guess what? Once they like you, they'll come back. That's the magic of building a relationship. Trust me on this one.

Cracking the Groupon Code

The key to making Groupon work for your business is to understand how to flip the insanely cheap price to your advantage. Don't think about today or tomorrow; think about the big picture.

Here's a concept that you'll get very familiar with in the permanent makeup industry: the long time value customer. This idea isn't actually limited to the permanent makeup industry, and can be applied to many different industries (so it's gainful concept to have in mind). Once this long time value customer walks into your shop and buys one procedure from you, the clock is ticking. It's your job to make her want to return to you—rather than someone else—for her touch-up.

Now let's put this into a marketing perspective. If you would usually need to pay 40% of your revenue to bring in a customer, Groupon actually works in the opposite direction. You're *getting paid* rather than *paying out* for advertising, and you're getting experience under your belt at the same time. See what I mean about the "no downside" part?

Let me give you a real-world example. Let's say you normally charge $800 for a microblading procedure, and you list it at 50% off with Groupon, bringing the first session down to $400. You've automatically got a happy customer on your hands. If you were to recommend an upgraded service such as Soft Ombré (for an additional $150), you'd barely have to talk about the fact that their brows would look a billion times better than just a normal microblading.

Can you guess how many women upgrade without a second thought? Tested by me, 99 out of 100 will add an extra service without batting an eyelash! And the best part? Those profits are all yours, baby. Groupon gets half of the microblading profits, but any upgrades or extras go straight into your pocket.

Then, this customer will return in 30 days for the first touch-up, and you better believe she'll pay you $300 for her dream eyebrows. At this point, it's your job as a smart businesswoman to touch up not only her eyebrows, but the relationship with her as well. Pick up where you left off. Talk to her. Make her want to come back to *you* next time, not the shop down the street.

Once you build a solid relationship with that customer, you can introduce new services and treatments. If the customer has trusted you with their face up to this point, you've earned status as their beauty guru. They'll trust you with pretty much anything. Whatever you recommend in order for them to look beautiful, younger, and more confident, they'll purchase. Eyeliner? No problem, do it. Plasma treatment? Yes please, whatever you say!

The biggest advantage to microblading is that each and every customer comes back once a year for a color refresh. This is just one more opportunity to offer services and treatments. Think of every single customer you will be bringing in with Groupon...now multiply that times once per year for a color top-off. You see where I'm going with this? The potential profits are insane.

Though Groupon may seem like you're losing money at first, take a look at the bigger picture. What you lose upfront, you more than make up on the back end. Patience is key. But then again, by this point in the book, you probably already knew I'd tell you to hold your horses and take your time.

Here's another tip I learned about pricing strategy: list high so you can discount low. When I say that, I mean that you need to list your price for microblading at a higher rate than what you actually charge, so that the customer feels like she's getting a discount. For example: I listed my microblading service at $300, but I charged $150. This made my clients feel like they struck gold, and it made them want to buy upgrade services from me. Peoples' responses will always be more positive when they see a discount or incentive—rather than just a cheap price—especially for a high-end service like microblading.

Another incredible way I booked so many clients (and still one of my favorite methods today) was by using half price/limited spots available ads on Facebook. Yes, that's right…I was advertising for free on social media, and don't think I had a marketing team with the latest and greatest tools. Oh no; it was just me, editing my own images in an app called Moldiv, cropping before and after photos of my clients.

Guess what? It freaking *worked*. Instantly, I had a line outside my beauty studio and I was waitlisting clients as far as three months out. Hear me when I say this: social media is one of the most powerful tools you can use to market yourself and your work.

And don't think I mean that you can just post a few boring photos on a Facebook wall and think that you're done. If it were that easy, we'd all be superstars, right? I'm talking about getting used to the idea of spending 40% of the money you make on promoting yourself.

I know, it sounds like a high number. It may sound crazy, stupid, and like a waste…and you probably want to shut the book right now after reading that. But listen to me. I started my multi-million dollar company with barely any money in my pocket. I've been there, done that. I know how hard it can be to get a business off the ground, and how frustrating it is when you're investing time and money in the wrong type of advertising.

Don't get overwhelmed by this. We'll jump back to advertising later in the book, and I'll outline exactly what you can do to market yourself like a pro to gain maximum exposure in the business world. There's no reason anyone should have to spend millions like I did—I can be the mentor that I wished I had had when I was just starting out.

One last tip for creating an audience with a small budget (but still important for optimal results) is to run contests. One of the most incredible marketing contests I've ever seen was the Dove Concept.

Dove's "Real Beauty Should Be Shared" contest on Facebook hit the branding bullseye. If you're not familiar with this contest, I'll sum it up: they ran a fill-in-the-blank contest with photos, asking fans to tell them how a friend represents "real beauty." The fan entered their friend in the contest by filling in the friend's name, as well as two things about the friend that make them beautiful.

In staying true to their brand, Dove didn't offer an iPad or some other type of extravagant prize. The winners of this contest got to become the next faces of Dove. Needless to say, this is a brilliantly-branded campaign. Not only did Dove get real, genuine faces for their in-store marketing campaigns, but their brand is further associated with real people and real beauty—not airbrushed models.

It gives life to their slogan and truly makes it more than just words.

You can follow this same concept with your microblading business. You don't have to be a huge company like Dove to copy this contest model. It's simple, just use Facebook. Try a contest like this: Tag 3 friends. Follow and Like this Page, and Share this Post for a chance to win a FREE microblading session.

Once you get that client in the door, build the relationship. Add the extra services. Touch up the color. Become their beauty guru. Congratulations, babe, you've gotten a long-term-value customer. Do the math. It always works out in your favor in the end.

Chapter 7
Doubled Discounts: Proven To Boost Sales Every Time

Objects In Motion Stay In Motion

This isn't just a law of physics—you can apply this principle to your business as well. Here's another real-life example from my past: about three months after I began offering microblading service in my shop, I booked my last few appointments for half price as a "Christmas offer."

When I took a look at just how much I had improved in only three months, I knew it was time to raise my prices. And when I say raise my price, I don't mean by just 5 or 10 percent. No, I *doubled* my price, but then I immediately switched back and discounted it again, offering a half-off discount.

Basically, my price was $300 per microblading service, but I was offering a half-off deal, so the cash-out price was $150. I doubled the original price, bringing the total to $600, but then switched gears and lowered the price again, bringing it back down for the customer to $300. Why did I do this? To level up, to gain authority, and be a little more selective about my clientele. Also, you can see now that I hit my target price of $300, and the customer felt like they were getting an exclusive deal.

Not only that, but I'll let you in on a secret: I figured I'd work less, since I was raising my prices. No such luck; I was still working my ass off 20 hours a day…I was just charging double. If I wasn't sleeping, at least I was padding my bank account pretty nicely, right?

I was still a newbie in the microblading game and under-evaluating my work, but check this out: in that three-month time span, I was quickly becoming one of the most well-known and best artists in Norway. Clients were flying in from Poland, Finland, and all over Europe to have me fix their eyebrows. Groupon gave me a huge leg up; with the profits I saved from those clients, I was able to not only pay my bills, but invest in paid advertising campaigns—building a pro website and preparing for the next level.

When I started raking in the big money, here's what I *didn't* do: I didn't run out to Jimmy Choo with my first big check. I didn't cash my windfall and blow it in the club on a Friday night. I mentioned before that I was a wife, a mom, and I don't hang out in the party scene anyway— but even so, do you know how I rewarded myself when I began to make real money? With a baguette. That's right: with bread. Now, I won't lie, it was a crazy-expensive BLT

Tuna Baguette (equivalent to around $20!), but that was enough for me. No big spending on fancy dinners, no flashy new handbags. Just a simple, delicious treat for hard work well done—and then it was back to the grind, baby.

After I secured my rotating base of core clients, I began to invest in business courses, learn about advertising, Search Engine Optimization (SEO), blogging, Instagramming, and all things digital media. Promoting myself online using those tools felt so foreign to me—after all, I had a law degree! And then I ran a beauty studio! But then I reminded myself of that very fact: I evolved from a lawyer to an aesthetician with zero knowledge or experience. If I could learn those skills, I could learn business and marketing, too. I'm always eager to teach myself new things, always on the hunt for new ways to grow.

And this is the key to why I have been so successful as one of the best artists in the world. As I said before, I couldn't draw a Christmas tree (and still can't)! A non-artistic lawyer *can* be the best with zero skills—the most important factor is to have an open mind and never stop learning. My goal was never to be an artist or to be able to sketch the perfect eyebrow—it was to follow a logic pattern and make millions.

But let me tell you something: making millions isn't everything, either. Now, I'm not saying not to shoot for the moon—you should absolutely do it. I can't imagine my lifestyle without private jets, oceanfront property, and being able to give my daughter the best care while enjoying 5-star accommodations all over the world. That's the dream, and I wouldn't trade it for anything.

What I mean is that the real addiction to my job came when I began to bring tears of happiness to my customers' eyes. My mission as an artist changed drastically, and so should yours. I became so thirsty to see people regain their confidence, to watch them undergo a transformation, and to bring them a happiness they didn't think they could feel when they looked in the mirror.

The best part of every treatment was always at the end—it was like a little dog wagging its tail as its owner stepped in the door after a long day at work—that kind of joy that I'd done an excellent job. And did I make everyone happy? Hell no—I'm not an avocado. But the point is that every day, I made sure to strive for maximum satisfaction.

No matter how exhausted I was, no matter how many hours my daughter kept me up the night before throwing a tantrum, no matter how tired my hands were, my customers came first. I never performed a procedure quickly just "to be done" with it. Take this mindset and use it to your advantage as well—never offer a service unless you can deliver the best out of it.

Just Say No

This is another valuable lesson I can teach you: the power of turning someone down. I learned this lesson the hard way (with tears of frustration), so take it from me: you are the artist, you have the education and qualifications, and you are the one who improves your customer's appearance. And, sadly, at the end of the day, your reputation is the one on the line...not your customer's. So say no to a customer if you feel that you can't satisfy their needs 100%.

This doesn't mean you're not good enough—don't get me wrong; you're brilliant. You're more than qualified, and you're an artist who is experienced, knowledgeable, and totally capable. But the reality is that you're not going to be able to make everyone on the planet happy. Why?

Because sometimes, a customer's expectations aren't realistic, or they simply don't align with your techniques.

Trust me on this: the money you turn away on that one client in the short term is nowhere near the amount of money you would lose if your name were tarnished by a mistake or a job done poorly. If you have one unhappy customer, that's an instant domino effect which seriously decreases your ability to gain new customers.

More often than not, your customers will respect and appreciate if you are honest with them upfront. Simply explain to them that unfortunately, you're unable to provide the service they request—due to the fact that you're not at the skill level required to perform the procedure.

Even if you are skilled enough, just let it slide. You know the old saying, *The customer is always right*? Well, it applies here. Let the customer believe that you're coming clean about something, let them feel like they have the upper hand. You're not in a position to tell the customer what's right or wrong, so just let them feel like they're in a position of power. Otherwise, they'll go right to their smartphone and bash you all over social media. And

POOF! Just like that, your reputation is on its way out the window, and you never even touched them.

The last thing you want is to "teach the customer a lesson"…even if you think they deserve it. Just be a pro, keep your business face on, and move along. One nasty person isn't worth your time, and surely isn't worth your reputation.

* * *

Don't compromise what you've learned when it comes to shape, color, and style. Customers' expectations normally don't reflect reality and what can actually be done to improve a person's eyebrows. The thing about a perfect microblading job is that when done right, everyone can tell—but at the same time, no one can tell.

What I mean by this is that perfectly microbladed brows look just that: perfect. No natural set of eyebrows can look that good, so clearly, work has been done to create that look. But on the other hand, a quality microblading job can't be detected because they look so natural.

It's the same concept with silicons. There are two types of customers: those who want to show off that they spent thousands of dollars, and those who want it to look natural and undetectable.

So if a client tells you during your consultation that she wants to have screaming eyebrows like two stamps on her face, she's not the customer for you. And really, she's not a good fit for microblading, either. Microblading is designed to improve the status of the eyebrows, correct small imperfections, define the shape, and create flawless, naturally beautiful arches. It's not meant to transform your entire face, change your features, or create drastic results...at least not in my world.

As an eyebrow guru expert, I can tell you the truth: if anyone looks at your eyebrows before they take a look into your beautiful eyes, then girl, you're in trouble. They're not looking at your brows because they are beautiful, they're staring at your brows because they're either too dark, screaming across your face, arched too high, or they just look fake. Eyebrows are the frame to the face—they should add expressivity to your eyes and outline your windows to the world—but they should *never, ever* scream that they look drawn on or fake.

I busted through the stigma that the practice of microblading is giving women fake eyebrows—yeah, at the end of the day, it's an illusion. But it's a far cry from the screaming stamps that others associate with "fake brows," and the results produced by microblading look so natural, that hardly anyone can tell the difference. For me, this isn't fake. It's as real as it gets.

Chapter 8
Skip The Spite, Play For Keeps

Don't Reinvent The Wheel

Needless to say, in another three months, I was doubling my prices yet again. Did I use the same strategy as before? You know it! Don't reinvent the wheel—this is a crucial strategy that I learned at this point.

So, let's take a look at the numbers: my original price went from $600 to $1200. Keep in mind that I wasn't actually charging these prices, just listing them on my menu of services to make the clients feel like they were getting a hot price. ("Grab that insane deal girl, it's 50% off!") I was actually charging half that—$300 per microblading session. When I doubled the price again, my "half-price" offer became my initial target of $600.

So, with that in mind, let's think about it like this: with every new client, I was becoming more and more of an expert in my field. You don't need a Masters degree in math to understand that in just 6 months, I was making six times what I started out charging—from $100 per microblading session to $600! I made a ton of money with nothing but the model I just shared with you—you're welcome!

I began to use my newfound social media skills more and more, posting my work day after day. Even if I noticed small imperfections; guess what? No one else did! I told you—I'm a perfectionist—what was obvious to my eyes went unnoticed by everyone else. In fact, with less than one year of experience in the microblading field, I was considered to be one of the best artists in the entire world. Yes, you read that right: me, with less than a year of practice under my belt, and I was one of the best on the planet.

I've seen it and microbladed it all: skin with large pores, scars, alopecia, clients with late-stage cancer, chemotherapy patients, customers with different types of diseases, female, male—you name it. As I gained experience in various situations, my skill set was undeniable, and my confidence became noticed by everyone around me.

Let's talk about what defines an *expert* for a moment. So often, people think that in order to become an expert in a certain field, you need to devote years of your life to it. Nope! Sixteen hours a day, every single day for a few months will beat 10 years with microblading as just a side hustle performing one procedure a month.

Guaranteed. If you're pouring your time and energy into your craft, it will reward you right back.

I was by far one of the youngest artists in the game, and I had to fight against my fair share of bullshit. *Oh, she is so new, her work is horrible!* Criticism like that from more seasoned artists followed me wherever I went, and I had to let it slide right off my back. Why? Because the work spoke for itself. When I looked down at really incredible work—eyebrows that looked beautiful, natural, and inspired women to go out and be their best selves—it always came from the hands of a younger artist.

The older generation of permanent makeup artists were (and sadly, still are) stuck in their ways. These "veteran" artists won't listen, won't evolve with the times, won't believe that trends change. They'll get in your face and scold you about how they learned to do eyebrows back when Christina Aguilera's black brows were hot, so don't try to tell them what to do.

In short, these older generation artists are stubborn and closed off to innovation. They're stuck in a rut and only shooting themselves in the foot from a business standpoint, because they refuse to take constructive criticism or understand the progress of their own industry. These are the types of people who put new artists down—the same spiteful people who discourage newbies by saying that microblading is a "talent" rather than a skill. Do yourself the biggest favor of all. Don't be like them. Skip the spite, and keep an open mind.

* * *

I doubled my price one more time with my special method, and then I kept my prices steady…with no discounts. Why would I suddenly change the game if I had been so successful in the past?

Let me answer your question with another question: have you ever seen Louis Vuitton, Hermès, Tiffany, or Cartier slap a discount sign out in front of any of their shops? Yeah, me neither.

That was me at this point. I was playing the high-end brand technique—I didn't discount my prices simply because *I didn't need to.* I had already hooked my clients, I was providing top-notch service, and they were going to shell out their money for it.

The next question you probably have is this: why wouldn't your clients just go somewhere cheaper? After all, if a person can't afford a Louis Vuitton bag, there are plenty of Gucci bags listed at 50% all the time. Why not switch to another qualified microblader that *does* offer a discount or a cheaper price?

This is the problem I faced. As I raised my prices and became more expensive by the day, I figured that I would lose a good chunk of my clientele. But, not to worry, because at this point, you should know that I found a way to combat that.

I went back into brainstorming mode, this time working to develop a new way to revolutionize the way microblading was performed. I created what is known today as a Soft Ombré effect—an upsell to my own Dual Blade Method of microblading—which took only 15 minutes of extra work and netted me an extra $300 per upgrade!

Not only was this a high-dollar upgrade (ka-ching!), but it significantly improved the final result of the microblading procedure for the client, which made it the most wanted service in the industry. At this point, I was a master in the field, and I had my customers' best interests at heart. I had developed a truly winning solution: not only was this a high-end upgrade, but honestly, one everyone needed. Like, *everyone.* Soft Ombré blends the strokes in such a natural way, it camouflages scars, it corrects old tattoos—I could go on and on. I'm so proud of this service that I could talk until tomorrow about it.

That passion spilled out into my sales pitch, and guess what? 99 out of 100 clients booked the upgrade without a second thought. And here's a little secret: for the one customer who said no…I'd be inclined to add it on for free. Why? Because it really is beneficial. It really does look ten times better than just a microblading session. And for just 15 minutes of extra work on my end, she feels like a VIP and tells all her friends. And that, baby, is free advertising.

Speaking of free advertising, this brings me to my next tip: whoever said a photo was worth a thousand words was wrong. It's worth much, much, more. If you take nothing else away from this book, just keep this in mind: photos are going to be your best methods to drive in revenue.

Your procedures are only ever as good as your photos. Remember that. You can perform the most beautiful procedure of your career, but if you take a photo with awful quality, you've done a bad job. The photos you post represent your brand, so you want to make sure that you're not harming your reputation by posting ugly photos and turning away customers before they ever even arrive.

Does this mean you need a fancy camera and Photoshop experience? Hell no! I never used anything more than an iPhone camera, and I believe you should never alter your photos in Photoshop. Clear photography at a good angle and quality lighting is all you need. It's priceless, in fact. This is your business card—spreading across the internet like wildfire.

Now, why shouldn't you use Photoshop? The answer is simple: you don't want to trick your customers. They're not stupid, and you shouldn't treat them like you're hiding something from them. If you edit your pictures or Photoshop redness away, you're only doing yourself a disservice. Be real. Be honest. Your clients will expect a little redness after the procedure—you're cutting into their skin, after all! There's nothing wrong with redness in an "after" photo, and you shouldn't have to Photoshop it away.

Another way to use media to your advantage: video. I created quick, ten-second clips of my clients after the procedure with a Q-tip running against the grain of their natural hair strokes. By doing this with the lens super-zoomed, you could get a glimpse at where the skin had been microbladed. To get an idea of what I'm talking about, check out World Microblading on Facebook and @worldmicroblading on Instagram.

You may be wondering how videos like these can help drive sales—well, they paid for some of the most luxurious holidays you can imagine. I'm not here to brag, I'm only here to educate. Like I said earlier, I used to be "in it win it," wanting nothing but a fat bank account and luxury beachfront bungalows, but my views have changed. I'm about helping people gain confidence, and spilling the secrets of what I knew to inspire legions of women across the world to rise up and achieve their own potential. After my inbox overflowed day after day with messages about how awesome my work was and questions about how I created this lifestyle, I knew it was truly time to take my skills to the next level.

Chapter 9
Lessons From The Breaking Point

From Microblader To Master Trainer To Multimillionaire

I developed a curriculum and began to teach small groups how to perform microblading procedures and of course—since I generally count progress in months rather than years—it didn't take me long to rise as one of the most acclaimed trainers in the world. And yet, at the same time, I'd soon come to be known as one of the most hated microblading artists on the planet by the competition...but more on that later.

What set me apart from other trainers was that I didn't see this as just a job. I cared about my students like I cared about my baby. I wanted to hold their hands, to guide them toward success; I never let them make a mistake. And yet, I was tough, raw, and mean at times; I saw tears of frustration—but in the end, I know I made a lasting impact on the lives of my students.

I saw many of them enter my training courses struggling to pay their mortgages, only to thrive in their careers as microblading artists, cashing out at $400,000 in a year. Yeah, that's right, four hundred grand *in a year.* I shared every single tip that I myself had learned and tested, and I wanted them to have the support and the confidence they needed to succeed.

In those days, I traveled frequently—I was back and forth between three different continents training students, serving my high-end clients, and overseeing my beauty studios. I was stretched thin, but I loved every moment. Again, I took it to the next level.

I kept improving my training programs, taking student feedback into account. I was already considered at the top of my game in microblading, and I was committed to rising to the top of education, too. And guess what? I did it. I raised the standards of training in microblading with every passing day.

I started out with 2- and 3-day training courses, but quickly dropped the 2-day course after realizing that this skill couldn't be taught in such a short span of time. It wasn't something I wanted to provide, and I felt like any course less than three days was putting my students at a disadvantage.

The 3-day with 1 live model course was born, and I supervised this totally hands-on class. In place of the 2-day course I scrapped, I created the 5-day intensive course with a minimum of three live models, which I always recommended as it was the much more economical deal. That course was so compressive that there was no way on Earth that you could leave without being able to perform a procedure from A to Z and produce the same results that I created after I squeezed over 20,000 eyebrows out of my hands.

Yeah, that's right: after my 5-day course, the novices were better-trained than I was when I was offering pro services in my beauty studio. This is when I first developed my 100% satisfaction guarantee—that if any student felt like they weren't adequately trained, their next course was free. I was *that* confident in my course's effectiveness.

It felt like I was working 25/8—every single day, Monday to Sunday, from early in the morning until I literally could not stay awake anymore. Once class was over, I was still engaged with my students; sharing my experiences and staying on the lookout with how I could help them grow and progress. Even though I was younger than most of my students, we'd still hang out after class. They'd take me to dinner at a place with incredible guacamole just because they knew I'd love it. Building a strong relationship with each student was one of my main goals. I wanted to be a part of their growth and their journey—I wanted to be remembered as the person who changed the course of their life forever.

I stayed humble during this time, not letting my status get to my head. I slept on the massage beds when I could catch a break in between the courses, and I'd dash to the airport to make my flight after each course was over...only to do it all over again in another city. I made decent money—I could afford to take things slow—but you know me well enough by now to know that I don't ever take things slow, now do I?

Here's where I'll dip into my personal story: as I mentioned before, I'm European. My training courses were taking place in the United States, and for my part, I lacked a lot of understanding about American culture as a whole. Specifically, in the summer of 2016, this ignorance came to bite me big time when these "veterans" of the permanent makeup industry saw the threat I posed to them.

What did these veterans of the industry do? Well, long story short, I refused to partner with them, and they got angry. Instead of just being mature about the denial, they reported me as an illegal alien to the American government—which ripped my world right out from under me. Everything I worked to achieve, everything I built for myself and my family…it was all gone. I lost my job, my right to visit the USA, and most importantly, my reputation.

I was sent back to Norway, deported from the United States at LAX—but you probably already know that I'm writing this book facing the Pacific Ocean from my place in Santa Monica. Because I took the hit at this early stage, I was given the authority to level up and beat out my competition in the long run.

I returned to Norway and got sucked into the most terrifying point of my life: a horrible divorce, my ex-husband trying to murder me, and then throwing my daughter and me out on the cold streets of Oslo in winter with no money, clothes, or food. I was the boss babe who had it all: the career, the husband, the lifestyle…and then I had nothing but $20 in my pocket and my autistic daughter in my arms—my beautiful, innocent child who had done nothing to deserve any of this.

My entire life was ruined at that point, and all because of social media. My ex teamed up with the most vicious wolves in the industry, and they ate me piece by piece. He claimed that he was the one who developed the Dual Blade Method. He stole my entire product line, and he tossed out restraining order after restraining order to gain control of my businesses (another lesson about being a foreigner in Norway…but that's reserved for my tell-all life story).

As I mentioned at the beginning, this book isn't about teaching you how to microblade. It's about life lessons, it's about learning to hustle, it's about taking examples from my life and using them to propel you forward in your own career. If there's any way for any of what happened to me to be useful, I want to use it to help and inspire the women around me.

And it can be useful, because guess what I learned? My ex tried every day of his life, in every single way, to take things from me…but you know what he couldn't take? My superpower. That's right. He claimed that he was the microblading expert, but check this out—I was still performing procedures, making a decent living, providing for my daughter (the same one he threw out on the street).

Even though my ex was spending every second of every day trying to tear me down, I was still working, still microblading, still using my superpower to my advantage. Why? Because at the end of the day, he could take my home, my food, my money, and even my clothes, but he couldn't take my superpower away from me. That was mine to keep, mine to nurture, mine to grow into something to push me forward into the prosperity of the rest of my life.

No matter what life throws at you or rips away from you, your superpower is always yours. Remember that.

I couldn't go back to the US, which stung me. Not only did I love it there, but it was the biggest market where there was the highest demand for expert trainers, and I was missing out on so much profit. But I had no other choice—I trained in different countries, avoiding the USA.

Microblading has saved me, time and time again, paying my bills and helping me to create what is today known as the largest microblading academy: World Microblading. If at the time that I created this company I *thought* I was pretty good at marketing…oh no, baby. I was mediocre.

I teamed up with a marketing guru and in less than three months at the start of 2017, World Microblading was already a multimillion dollar business—a legit academy with a few trainers working under my close supervision. I was still living in Oslo at this time, and I flew my top trainers to me to teach them every secret possible in order to surge their success in the US market. As a result, we absolutely crushed the competition, and we scaled on a level that no one could compete with. We blew our competition out of the water, and we did it by doing things with proven marketing strategies.

Chapter 10
Making Your Mark

Making Marketing Work For You

After watching my company blow itself into such a rapid success, I took a hard look at what I did differently this time around. I was successful when I marketed myself in my beauty studios, but the level of success that I saw with World Microblading was insane. I wanted to understand what caused such a big difference in results, so I examined my own actions.

And here I started to understand what real marketing means—what it means to invest millions in ads, tests, excellent SEO, an amazing website, graphic designers, user experience engineers, a development team, and so much more. I started to understand each element of the team, and how important each aspect was in order to scale a business. I was at the top of the microblading game and I had street smarts for days, but let's face it, I was far from what you'd call a professional marketer or a CEO. On top of that, my useless law degree didn't help.

I educated myself, I joined masterminds, I surrounded myself with bright business-focused people who helped me to level up. The price doubling of a microblading procedure seemed like common sense to me, but taking a business from seven figures to eight figures is pretty complicated—trust me. You're in a new league of scaling, and even though the basic principles are the same...you've got so much more on your plate in terms of PR, advertising, branding, and marketing. I could scale a business from five to six figures in my sleep. Six seven figures was bearable (with a lot of work), but from seven to eight wasn't easy. In fact, I've poured over $65,000 in just the past few months into continuing to educate myself so that I could provide more and more insight to our students.

Here's what got to me the most: after training thousands of students, I was still frustrated that not all of them were unlocking their potential. Don't get me wrong— my students were making good salaries (there's really no way to fail as a microblading artist...unless you're incredibly lazy and don't bother to change out of your pajamas before work).

But I couldn't figure out why my students weren't scaling past just decent money. I'm talking about hitting a five-figure income; why only a few of them were going on to cash out at $200k, $300k, or $400k in the year 2017...

and then it hit me. These students didn't want to do the extra work that it takes to hit a five-figure salary.

Remember, to hit five figures, you need to make just under $8400 per month. Yeah, you read that right. $8,333 x 12 months = $100,000—you do the math.

Now, can you achieve this? Of course you can. But we've got to talk about marketing...and I've got to warn you that you need to keep an open mind about testing. Just because a certain type of marketing works for your neighbor, it doesn't necessarily mean it will work for you.

First tip: start small, but keep a generous budget on hand for advertising. If you want to scale fast, invest 80% of how much you make in profits right back into your marketing. You'll be amazed at how fast your business takes off.

Word-of-mouth is great, but it's not everything. It's not going to take you to the next level. It'll bring you a few customers for sure, but if you want to scale up fast, you're going to have to invest in proper advertising.

I said it before and I'll say it again: the minimum investment in advertising is 40% of your income. This is

NON-NEGOTIABLE. Trust me on this one—you'll thank me later after your business surges. And if you're not willing to hear me out on this, well, then you might as well stop reading now. Trash this book and you eat an ice cream, because you're wasting your time otherwise.

* * *

At the time of this book's writing, it's 2018. If you don't have a website, you live under a rock...and you're shutting out good business. Get yourself a decent website that looks professional and aesthetically pleasing. Let's take a look at the website I had when I was a microblading artist in Norway: www.microbladingoslo.com.

Right off the bat, you can see that the domain name is simple, clear, easy to remember, and awesome for your SEO. Moving forward, there should be things on the main page that you should never skip. For instance, every professional website should always be crisp, fast, and simple to navigate.

Here's something important: if someone approaches you to say that they can design a beautiful website for you for a thousand bucks...politely turn them down. Save your money babe, I can guarantee you that website will be down every other day, take forever to load, and probably look extremely boring. In all honesty, you'd most likely drive away your clients before they even book the service with you.

Prepare to drop $4,000 to $5,000 on a quality website with a beautiful design and and a $500 monthly maintenance fee at the minimum. This will set you apart from your competition and make your business stand out among all the others in the crowd. How so? You'll have expert speed optimization, sharp SEO, a graphic design team to craft a beautiful logo for your company, a copywriter to assist with offers...the list goes on and on.

Once your pro website is all set up with a professional logo, vision for your company, mission statement, and content, make sure that you have your business's details clearly visible for your customers to see. You want to have aesthetically-pleasing graphics on display with a full address, a detailed menu of services listed, testimonials, before and after photos, as well as a description of each service that you offer. Most importantly, you want to include an online booking system right there on your website—make it easy for your customer!—and make sure that the booking system automatically links with your digital calendar.

Next step: trash the regular calendar on your agenda. It's not going to work for you when you hit the big leagues. If you have 10 clients per day, you're going to get overwhelmed and you will mess up. With a professional booking system, you get built-in help to send your clients email reminders, appointment confirmations, and you already have the information you need to build an email list (which is a goldmine...but more on that later). In addition, you can even charge a deposit to secure a booking reservation.

Here's a clear example you can use for a website model that's been tested for maximum success.

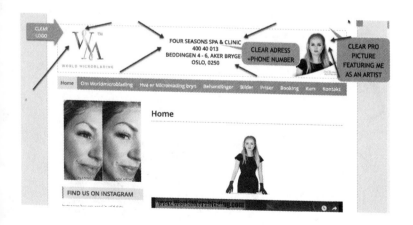

You can see right there in the picture: a winning website should feature a clear photo of you or your business, the contact details, and the logo. All these elements should pop out, clear and visible, from the very first moment someone clicks onto your page. You have about two seconds for a potential client to decide whether or not they want to grab a lead before either closing the page or moving forward. Yes, two seconds. So in those two seconds, you need to sell yourself, your skill, and your business, and make this person decide to book a service with you. Make those two seconds count.

After you've got an eye-catching front page, create the following options.

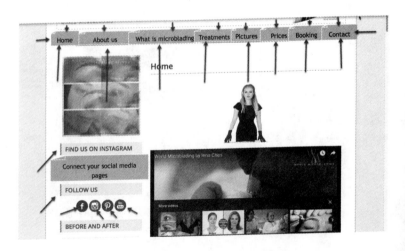

Every single rubric is essential to creating the elements of a professional website. They all work together to form one complete site, so it's important not to skip any of these tabs.

On your Home page, you should have a video of you performing a microblading procedure, which will grab the attention of the client right away. Here's the thing: many of our clients aren't really sure what microblading is. It may seem strange, but they think they're getting hair plugs or some other kind of unrealistic procedure—don't judge, educate. It's best to remember that the clients are paying you their hard-earned cash for the service, so the more information you have on your website now, the less headache you'll have later. You do the work upfront to create it, and it stays there forever.

Now, back to the video: not only will it educate your customers, but video footage has been proven to grab a customer's attention over 400 times more than a simple photo.

Needless to say, a video comes in pretty handy when you need to make two seconds count!

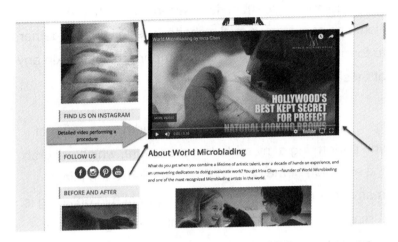

Moving forward—how are you branding yourself? Who are you, what authority do you have in the microblading business, and why should your customer pay *you* an insane amount of money instead of your

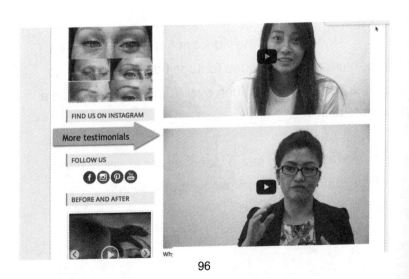

neighbor down the street (who's charging half price)?

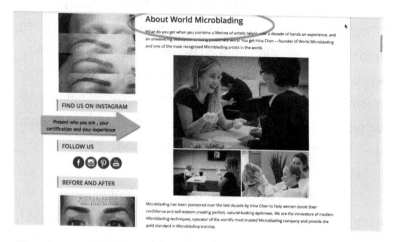

Check this out:

As you can see, even though I was (and still am) at the top of the microblading game, I used the brand World Microblading to level up. It's a huge, international academy with a top-notch reputation and even though I'm a great artist with an authority in the industry, I want that extra power that my brand can buy. I want to use the brand's authority, and you can too.

It's so important to have the backing of a big company and use it for your advertising. When you connect with that brand, you're associating yourself with that company's excellence.

On your own website, add a line that states "Trained By: ..." and place a picture with you, your trainer, and your certification details. No one wants to have their eyebrows done by someone who learned how to microblade on Youtube. Customers do their research when they look for a microblading artist—believe me—and they will know if you're legitimately trained.

It may seem difficult to get your foot in the door to microblading. Hear me when I say this: it's okay to be new, as long as you tie yourself to a large brand. Use their reputation and method as your backing, and you'll be just fine.

Next up on your website: include testimonials. This will help your audience trust you without ever coming face to face with you.

As I mentioned earlier in the book, before and after pictures are a must. The customer needs to understand what you're doing, and this is the best way to educate them outside of creating a video.

And then, top it off with even more testimonials. This really hits it home that you're providing a service that is top-notch and high-quality.

Every single section needs to be treated with maximum care and consideration. We live in a world now where people will just book things online—90% of my customers never called or sent an email—so your site needs to be at the top of its game. Don't leave anything up to chance. Don't let anyone get away. The money is there—all you have to do is grab it.

Chapter 11
Outsource and Optimize

When In Doubt, Delegate It Out

So, your clean, professional website is up and running, enticing new clients to book with you each day. That means you're done with this step in the process, right?

Think again! You're just getting started. Even though your website is beautifully designed and your information is out there forever, the site itself will need monthly maintenance for thing like updates, speed optimization, and any kind of technological advancement. You want to always be on the cutting edge, and you always want to be at the top of your game.

I know what you're probably thinking at this point: *How am I supposed to know everything about web design and SEO while I'm supposed to be focusing on doing an awesome microblading job for my clients?* Here's the biggest little secret I know, a secret that has made my life ten million times easier over the years: don't take on every job yourself.

Yeah, that's right. You don't have to be superwoman. This is where teamwork comes into play.

One of the best things I ever did for myself and my business was to outsource all my tasks to a team of specialized professionals—not only was I taking the stress of each task off my own shoulders, but I was assigning tasks to professionals who could perform these tasks much better than I could. My company flourished, and in turn, grew substantially! Oh…and did I mention the fact that my life got insanely easier once I made this small switch?

At this point, I pretty much outsource my entire life. I don't even book my own flights or take my clothes to the dry cleaners—that's how addictive delegation has become for me! This is the key to succeeding in your business: using your time wisely. If you are wasting your time on tasks that take up too much of your precious time, then you need to find a different strategy to manage how you're spending your day. The old saying *"Time is Money"* has stuck around for good reason…because it's true!

So, how do you go from superwoman doing it all to savvy delegator? First things first: build a strong base team of professionals to handle your core needs. Once you have this foundation team to take care of things like web design and SEO, you can move on to smaller things like the daily tasks I mentioned above.

The Power of SEO

Search Engine Optimization (SEO) may seem like just a meaningless acronym, but don't mistake this powerful tool for something useless. In today's digital world, it's priceless to have a killer SEO strategy to drive clientele to your website in order to boost your bookings.

Now, let me ask you this: are you an SEO expert? Because I'm not. I would say I'm a great visionary, and strategist, and I can really do deep brain work, but I'm not a strong implementer. This is another reason why I choose to outsource—I love the fact that I can create the strategy, vision, and goal...then outsource the smart tech brains to implement it. See what I mean?

As much as I preach self-education, hear me when I say this: the smartest thing you can do for your business is to have an expert take control in this area of your business. This is where you need to take a step back and hire in an SEO consultant to work his or her magic for you, because (trust me on this one), they will do a *much* better job than you.

At this point, you're probably wondering what SEO actually does for you, and why it's so important. Basically, Search Engine Optimization is the process of maximizing the number of visitors to a particular website by ensuring that the site appears high on the list of results returned by a search engine. The key to getting more traffic to your website (which will obviously lead to customers) lies in integrating content with SEO and top-notch social media marketing (and we will get there shortly).

So what does all this mean in regular English? Think about it like this: when you move to a new city and you need to find a place to have your nails done, what's the first thing you do? You Google nail salons, of course. Think of some of the words you might use for the search bar in Google. You'd probably search for "best," "top," "awesome," "nail salons," as well as the city where you live, or maybe the neighborhood where you're located. These keywords are what SEO experts use to determine what drives customers to certain websites, and when done properly, it can pinpoint your target customers directly to your site. Pretty cool, right?

Now, with quality SEO and proper marketing work done, you're going to rank in Google pretty fast—especially if you're located in a top market like NY, LA, or DC. Keep in mind that "pretty fast" doesn't necessarily mean "overnight," though—this is a process. Just like there's no diet pill that will cause you to drop 50 pounds in one day, the same principle applies here. Realistically speaking, you'll be looking at a few months of hard work, dedication, perseverance, and patience, especially if you don't live in a big city. But if there's anything we've learned so far, it's this: if it were easy, everyone would be successful, right?

In my experience, I knew that teaching myself SEO would require way too much time and effort that I really couldn't spare. It was never my strength or my passion...I just knew I wanted my business to be at the top of the list when someone searched for microblading on Google. And guess what? After delegating that job to the experts, voilà! World Microblading was popping up first thing on Google search results every time.

If you randomly search "microblading training," here's what you get:

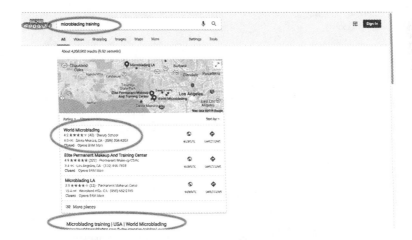

Now, you can see from the photo in the previous page that World Microblading is number one in both the organic search as well as number one in the map search. This is when you're searching across Google as a whole— notice that I didn't make any mention of my own business or California—just microblading. But because my SEO is so strong, Google was able to pinpoint my specific search terms exactly toward World Microblading.

But that's not all SEO can do for you. Check this out:

I randomly searched "microblading training Washington DC," and guess what? The first two links in the organic search are us! The Maps suggestion as a

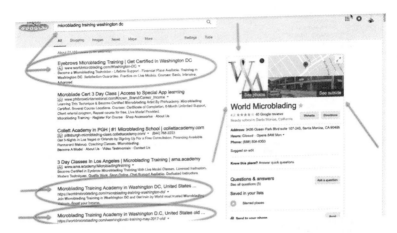

trusted business in Google suggests our academy. How did we make this happen? The power of SEO, babe.

Let me point out something else. Take a quick look at the screenshot again.

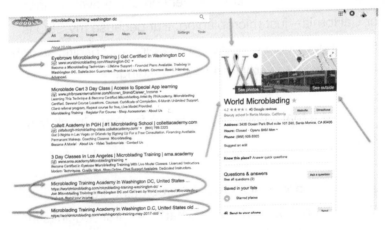

Notice that we are the first ad directly underneath the search bar, and there are three other competitors— below us, of course. But *why* are they below us? Because money talks, in a nutshell. When you want to be on the top of a paid ad, be prepared to shell out big money. We outbid all our competition and offered the highest amount of money to Google in order to maintain our position at the top of the paid ad content.

Think about it. How many times have you scrolled down past more than five links to find what you're looking for, no matter what it is: meal prep, diet, microblading training, manicure near me? I'm telling you—almost never. Ninety percent of the time, you're going to go with one of the top three links suggested by Google. Why? Because Google is your friend, girl!

Now let me ask you this: how often do you go digging onto page 2 or 3 of your Google search results? Have you ever even looked at page 2 or 3? Personally…I only dig that deep when I'm looking for my poor competition…just to check on them and see how they're doing back there. (Trust me, you don't want to be in that place. I can tell you from experience—I wouldn't be here today if I hadn't learned some hard life lessons from my spot on Page 2 of Google's search results, that's for sure.)

Again, one of the most important things is to know what you don't know. I knew that I didn't understand SEO, but I knew that I could delegate these tasks to a pro and have them done with precision. Did it work? You tell me! Go ahead, start Googling. The results speak for themselves.

Here's the main takeaway: proper SEO is going to cost you upfront. Hiring a team of professionals is, of course, going to take some money out of your pocket at first. But don't see it as a drain on your finances. It's essential to view this as an investment—because that's exactly what it is. SEO can make or break your business, and when done right, it can save you millions on advertising.

Remember when I said I didn't rush out to Jimmy Choo when I started making money? Use that same principle now. Don't reward yourself with a new pair of shoes or a gorgeous handbag when the money rolls in. Pour it right back into your business. Reward your efforts with better SEO strategies and targeted marketing. You'll thank me later.

Chapter 12
That App You're Browsing? It Can Make You Rich.

A World In Your Pocket

We live in the most incredible time for advertising that has ever existed: a time when pretty much everyone on the planet carries around a little advertising device right in their pocket, purse, or in the palm of their hand. That's right: smartphones and social media are the key ways to reach an audience on a large scale.

Once you have your website with targeted SEO in order, you need to move on to social media. Personally, I use Facebook and Instagram as my main tools. Over the past few years, I've spent millions advertising on these platforms, testing out different strategies and learning the industry from the inside-out. It's through this knowledge that I've established myself as a social media guru—in fact, one of my other businesses teaches women how to make money through social media marketing, empowering them to gain financial independence. I've created an incredible community from the ground up at www.fablifesociety.com, which I'm pretty proud of, if I do say so myself.

Enough about my social media credentials, though, here's how you can use these amazing tools your advantage in business. The first thing you need is a Facebook Business Page. *Please* do not use your personal Facebook page—get a professional one. Here are the very basic first steps to creating your Facebook Business Profile.

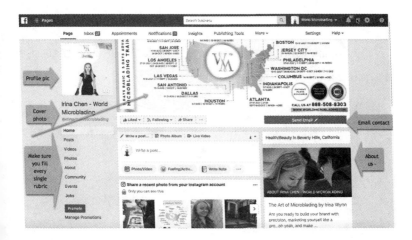

       Make sure you're taking advantage of every single rubric. The last thing you want is for a potential customer to have to scroll for five minutes to find your phone number, your website, or your email address. Remember what I said about the two-second rule on your website? Keep that in mind here, too. You want your profile to hold someone's attention, and the last thing you want is for them to give up and exit out of your page because they can't find what they need.

Also, make sure your walls are clean and full of valuable content. Be sure to use correctly-sized images for your profile picture and cover photo and to make sure that they're centered properly. You want to give off a professional image, so make sure to post photos to showcase that.

Your About section comes next. When completed, it should look like this:

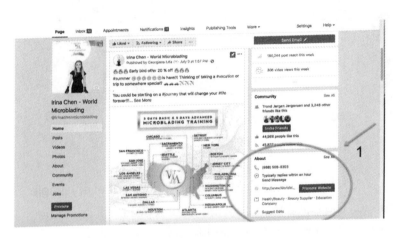

This is very simple, and all the fields should be easy fill in. Make sure that you reply to messages quickly so that Messenger will list you as a rapid responder. Your potential customers will notice this, and trust me—it makes a huge difference when someone is looking for a quality microblading artist. They are paying their hard-earned money to get microbladed—and they don't want to wait! Especially for a high-end service like this, their excitement is likely to fall with every minute you don't respond to their message on Facebook.

Too busy performing microblading procedures to wait by the phone and answer messages? No problem. When in doubt, delegate it out, baby.

When To Post, What To Post, and How Often Should You Post?

These are the most common questions when it comes to posting on a Facebook business profile, and I'm here to answer them. Here are your main objectives: to maintain a positive vibe and to keep your audience interested in your product.

So, how do you do it? First things first: post high-quality photos—only the best. Never, ever post a crappy photo, because that's going to de-legitimize your brand. You want to associate your business with quality and excellence, so you want to make sure that the type of content you post is top-notch.

The next rule of thumb: do not over-spam. Your goal is to connect with your followers, not bug them. Don't post just promotional content only, keep a good balance of content. For example, toss in a few inspirational quotes with service specials, maybe some gorgeous photos you took yourself to mix things up. The goal is to keep your feed balanced so that it your customers are engaged when they look at it, not bored. You want to share media with your audience (and sprinkle some ads for your services too get their minds working in the right direction), not bombard them with ads for your business.

So, how often should you post? Every day is optimal, but limit it to once—maybe twice. Once you reach three posts a day, you're walking into spam territory, and that's a surefire way for your followers to mute you, unfollow you, or just scroll past your posts in their feed. Plus, with so many different features in social media, the Feed isn't really the time or the place for multiple posts per day—that's where Stories are your friend (but more on that later).

As you can see from the screenshot on the next page, using emoticons is a way to grab attention fast.

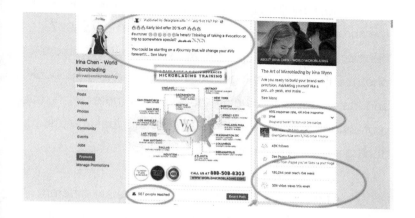

Also, it adds a personal touch to your post and helps you interact with your audience, so I always recommend that you place appropriate emoticons in a post. They engage with an audience in a way that I've never seen before.

Allow yourself to draw inspiration from your competition, but be original. Keep your integrity, and don't copy anyone's marketing style. I have zero respect for plagiarism attempts, and neither should you. Remember, you are the voice of your business…so make sure that your voice is an honest one.

Now, moving along; you can see at the bottom of the screenshot that this photo I posted "reached" 987 people. This means that I got 987 views on just this one photo! This is why having a business profile on Facebook and Instagram is so crucial—not only is it more professional, but you receive data like this that you just don't get from a personal account!

When you're promoting an ad, there are different types of promotions you can use in Facebook: you can either promote a service, create an offer, run a content, or point people in the direction of your website. Based on what you're focused on promoting, you want to be sure that you're sending your customers to the specific link that takes them where they should go. For example, this can either be an offer or a service, but don't just drop them on your website and have them figure it out for themselves— make the navigation easy for them. Pinpoint them in the exact location where they need to go.

As I mentioned before, videos are amazing at capturing your audience's attention. So are before and after photos, which go hand-in-hand with the way offers and contests pop on Facebook. When you're creating your ad, make sure you phrase it in a way that sounds irresistible. Also, make sure it looks clean, that it delivers all relevant information, and that it's capped off with a call to action ("learn more") button at the end. This drives traffic to your promotion and gets your audience excited.

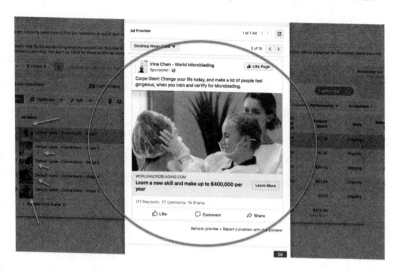

    On the left-hand side, you can see examples of ads we're testing out to measure which ones are performing better than others. This is pretty advanced marketing strategy, but if you want to go big—you'll either have to learn this yourself or outsource it to someone who can handle this for you.

    In my opinion, Instagram is an even more powerful tool for marketing and advertising than Facebook. It's my personal favorite—if only for the fact that Stories are such a popular feature. This is a revolutionary way to interact with your audience and share content, allowing you to post multiple times per day without spamming your followers.

Instagram Stories create relationships with your customers by giving them a chance to follow your journey and relate to you. Your potential clients want to see your procedure from start to finish, and they're interested in what's going on behind the scenes. Stories give them a glimpse into what's going on in your studio—giving potential customers an inside look at before, during, after the procedure, and all the steps in between.

Stories are for more than just posting about your procedures (which, of course, brings exposure to your business); you can actually advertise in a story! And here's the kicker: when you have a business account on Instagram with over 10k followers, you unlock the "swipe up" feature, which means that you can insert a call to action directly in a story post. That's just one fewer step for your followers to take in order to get where you want them: your website.

When you're posting on your business's Instagram account, you want to keep a clean persona with crisp walls full of the very best content you can find. This material should be inspirational and uplifting—keeping that positive vibe to elevate the mood of your clients—and post multiple times a day on this platform. My personal favorite times are 7AM and around 12:30PM. Why these times? That's when people are headed to work and on their lunch breaks—two of the tested and proven times that most people are scrolling through their phones.

Here's something to keep in mind: clients don't actually care about your product. Yeah, I know, it feels like a punch in the stomach to read, but the sooner you admit it, the more successful your business will be. The truth is that customers have marketing pushed in their faces from literally every direction—all day every day. All they really want out of microblading is the end result: how you can impact their life, bring value to it, and revitalize their confidence. At the end of the day, your clients want to feel beautiful, sexy, bold—and they want someone to get rid of their shitty eyebrows.

They don't really care about the actual process. All customers really care about are a few key factors:

- *Is my artist competent enough to trust with my face?*

- *Is my artist certified by a reputable microblading academy?*
- *Is this person posting quality before and after photos on their portfolio? Do I like their style?*
- *Does (s)he use sterile tools?*
- *Does (s)he use top quality products on my face?*
- *How much does the service cost? Is this person in my budget?*

After all these boxes are checked in the minds of your prospective clients, they're going to want to book a time slot with you. Because yes, you're tattooing eyebrows—but that's only what you're doing on the surface. What you're really doing is restoring hope, rebuilding confidence, and renewing a sense of empowerment for those who haven't felt beautiful in weeks, months, or even years.

I've worked with customers who were too shy to sleep next to their husbands without a full face of makeup on—even if they'd been married for 20 years! Yeah, that sounds insane, but it's true. In my experience, I've worked with customers who had alopecia, cancer, and other types of illnesses that took away their hair permanently...and guess what? Microblading was able to restore their confidence in a way they never anticipated. I've seen women cry tears of joy just from being able to feel beautiful again, especially after a sickness has ravaged their body. You really have no idea how dramatically two little strips of hair can change someone's life until you're in this industry, giving women hope where no one was able to give it to them before. And once you build that bond, you've created a lifetime customer.

* * *

At the end of the day, no matter how skilled of an artist you are, you're going to need a marketing team that's just as good...if not better. Just like I said at the beginning of this book: so many bright artists fade out and never get noticed—why? Because no one knows who they are! Don't let that happen to you. Don't let all your hard work, education, and skill go to waste. Marketing is expensive, it's difficult, it takes time, and it takes patience. But look where it gets you.

Right now, just over the brim of my laptop, the sun is setting over the waves of the Pacific Ocean in my "front yard." Still think it's not worth it?

Chapter 13
Utilize Lists and Level Up

Email Lists: A Goldmine

Remember how a few chapters back I said that an email list is crucial to your success? An email list is basically your net worth. You should build a list by having people subscribe to a newsletter you send out. You can collect information from your customers as soon as they visit your website, then import the data into your booking system and then into a Customer Relationship Manager (CRM) platform to send emails. Each day that you're not sending out emails, you're losing money.

So, you should be sending out offers every day, right? Wrong. If you spam out ads for your business every single day, your clients are going to lose interest fast. Worst of all, you'll come across as desperate. Instead, send tips about beauty, blog posts about what's new in the industry, and any kind of relevant info you have that your customer would want to read.

Make sure that 1 in 10 emails is an offer, and stay consistent. Send out emails around twice a week, on popular days like Tuesday and Friday. These are proven to have the highest opening rate and will get you the most optimal results.

Make sure that you're using catchy subject lines and emoticons and coupons. This way, your opening rate will dramatically increase. Also, use language that conveys a sense of urgency; phrases like "ends tonight," "just announced," or "last spots available." When you use this type of language, it makes your customer jump at your ad and react immediately.

Make sure you're adding clear call to action buttons on your emails which direct your customers to your website in order to book their services. No one wants to hunt around to book anything, and if you've got your customer's attention, the last thing you want is to lose it because they're confused about where to go or how to give you money.

Another thing to consider is to run specials for holidays. Thanksgiving Day, Black Friday, Women's Day, Mother's Day—you name it—these are all important celebrations, and people are generally in a festive mood. You can cash in on that by taking advantage of the holiday and driving the customers right into your doors.

And the benefits don't stop with an email list, either. Having a phone number list is another huge asset that you can take advantage of to drive your customers in for appointments. Send offers twice a month, but be sure not to overdo it on the phone calls or texts. You don't want your customers to only book with you when you have an offer for them.

Here's an awesome example of a text message you want to shoot out (which highlights all the key points of what you're trying to stress to the customer):

50% off this Friday for Microblading, LAST CHANCE to book, only 1 spot left. Text me back if you'd like to reserve your spot. Deal ends tonight at 8:00PST.

When you place deadlines and scarcity words in your promotional texts, your customer feels a sense of urgency, and is more willing to book with you right then. Scarcity words are phrases like, "only one spot left" and "limited space appointments available." Deadlines can be phrased like, "deal ends tonight at 8:00PST." When people feel the heat of a lifetime opportunity slipping through their fingers, they're much more likely to commit.

Now, when you're sending out your text message correspondence, you want to have a streamlined message that matches your email list promotions. Before you send out messages, have a clear vision of what you want to say and how you want to say it—ideally with tested marketing analytics to back you up—and then distribute it on all channels. Don't just make something up.

And, most importantly, before you set up any email or phone list whatsoever, invest in the smartest invention of them all: an automated system that removes people who have unsubscribed. Why? Because the last thing you want when you're trying to make millions is to be slapped with a lawsuit, that's why.

Leveling Up And Extending Your Reach

We covered the basics of setting up your social media and posting every day—now it's time to gain a massive amount of followers. After all, what better way is there to get noticed in this day and age than a free app that pretty much everyone is addicted to?

The easiest way for you to level up on social media is to get more followers, plain and simple. You need to get your product out there, and the best way to do that is to reach out to influencers to promote it. Your first step is going to be to reach out to "up-and-coming" influencers—these include accounts that have only 30k-50k followers. Make sure the followers aren't fake, and after you've vetted the account holders to ensure they're legit, go ahead and reach out by offering them a service for free in exchange for a post about your business. Simply shoot them a message or an email (both, even, to make sure that they see your request) and start a friendly dialogue with them, asking if they'd be interested in a free microblading session in exchange for some promotion. The worst that can happen is that they say no, or ignore you. Big deal.

You'll notice that I was specific about "up-and-coming" influencers with no more than 50k followers... there was a reason for that. Normally, social media influencers with more followers than that have PR agencies working on their behalf and require payment per post. Here's the thing, the small influencers aren't really going to blow your business up. They're a good stepping stone, but not a final measure. In order to get your business the attention it deserves, you're going to have to pay a legitimate influencer.

These top influencers (those with around 100k followers) and their PR firms come with a high price tag—but I can tell you from experience that they're well worth it. They interact with an engaged crowd much more so than a smaller social media presence can. When I say "high price tag," what do I mean, exactly? To reach followers in the triple digits, prepare to pay anywhere between $8,000 and $15,000.

Now you have to ask yourself: is this price worth it for you? It probably is. Think about it: you'll end up with promotional materials, and the content will be posted on this influencer's social media wall, attracting customers all the time.

A few words of warning: be sure that you are the legal owner of the content you provide to the influencer, and require that the type of post is permanent. For example, make sure the influencer doesn't add your post to his or her Story instead of a Wall post, because Story posts disappear after 24 hours. If you're shelling out thousands of dollars to reach followers, you want your content to stay put!

So, is this a wise choice to do first thing? Hell no. Don't rush out and pay a top influencer with your first big paycheck—even though that's better than blowing it on bottle service at a nightclub. Keep your head on your shoulders, and be patient. Paying a top influencer is a step I recommend only when you've got at least 200 clients in your rotation and your business is booming. Otherwise, you can use a multitude of other tactics without having to resort to spending that kind of money.

As I said before, use small influencers as a stepping stone. Reaching out to a 70k follower account, in my personal experience, might bring you around 2-5 new customers—which is well worth it in the long run. Never feel like you're cheating yourself or your business by offering a service for free; see it instead as a marketing cost. At the end of the day, the influencer is creating content and advertising your business in exchange for your work. And what's more: you had better work your ass off, because that Instagram influencer, beauty blogger, or Youtube star is going to write up a review of your service which will ultimately help drive your SEO. Do you see where I'm going with this? Sure, you're "giving away" a microblading service, but what you're getting in return is so much more valuable.

One final tip on leveling up: if you can swing it, try to book a spot on a newscast. I'll be honest, this is pretty unlikely if you don't have a top-notch PR team at your disposal, but if there's one thing I advocate, it's to try something until someone tells you no…and then try again a different way.

Television, like video clips on your website, is one of the most effective ways to capture someone's attention and help them understand your business. Start small by trying to land spots on local news stations, and work your way up from there. As I've mentioned before, so many people are either confused about the microblading process, or completely in the dark about it. By educating people about what it is that you do, you can brand yourself as an authority figure in a way that blows your competition straight out of the water. Your clients will not only flock to you, but they'll choose you over and over again, guaranteed.

Chapter 14
What Not To Do

Whatever You Do, Never Settle

It was a truly bittersweet point in my career when I realized that I in order to charge more, I needed to offer my customers an additional service. I wanted to maintain a higher cash flow, but I also wanted to keep my clients happy—so I set to work. It took me months of thinking and testing, but I finally developed my Soft Ombré effect which is still one of the most recommended add-ons to microblading service. It became a leader in the market as far as upselling was concerned—benefitting both the clientele and the business substantially. It was one of the best services I could have possibly come up with the upsell, and later led to the development of lash enhancement and lip tattooing.

Here's the main thought: you always want to be on the cutting edge. Never let a trend pass you by, and never, ever, *ever* settle. Always educate yourself on what's happening outside your own bubble, and stay current on what's happening inside your industry, too. Because guess what? If you're not going to provide these types of services, someone else is more than willing to step in and do the job.

At this point in the book, I've talked extensively about all the things you should do to help grow your skill set, your business, and your social media presence. I want to flip the coin now and warn you about some things you *shouldn't* do if you want to scale and be productive.

1. Don't take shortcuts when it comes to education.

Yes, it's going to cost less to attend a lower-quality institute for your microblading certification, and yes, you can just recycle that money back into your company. But should you do that? *Hell no!* Building a solid foundation of the concept of microblading is crucial to your success. When you skimp on proper training, it's like building a house out of old, rotting wood instead of the firm, sturdy bricks of a hands-on, quality guarantee of a reputable company. Get certified by the best of the best. Always remember: you get what you pay for.

2. Don't be lazy—go all in or just stay home.

If you think that you can cut corners and race your way to the top, I hate to be the one to burst your bubble...but you're wrong. You've got to put everything into this. You've got to be willing to sacrifice your nights, your weekends, your family time, your "me time." You have to visualize your financial goals and drive yourself toward them relentlessly. You have to dedicate your entire life to building your business, your brand, and your skill set. There's a reason that only a select few people on this planet are successful; it's because success is bought with patience, sacrifice, and hard freaking work.

3. Don't lose yourself in the details. As much of a perfectionist as I am when it comes to the microblading procedure (and you should be too), I learned that life isn't always smooth sailing. Sometimes, you have to just let things go. Trust me, you'll save yourself so much time and energy by learning to let go. Not sure if an ad is good? Test it out, and take a look at the analytics. If it does poorly, let it go…even if you loved it. Remember: you advertise based on what the customer likes, not what you like.

Case in point: when choosing the cover for this book, I opened a Platinum contest on <u>99designs.com</u>. After selecting 10 top-notch designs created by some of the best artists, I made a pool where I asked the audience for their opinion on which of the ten cover designs was their favorite. My personal favorite cover ranked number seven out of 10…pretty mediocre, if you ask me. I didn't understand how, though; my favorite was gorgeous, with all the elements of a cover that I wanted to present for my debut book. The details were subtle and elegant, the colors were striking yet chic...I absolutely adored this design. And still, it came in as number seven.

I wasn't convinced, though. I created another pool, this time limiting the choices to five covers (but including my favorite, of course, despite the fact that it ranked number seven in the previous pool). This top-five pool was limited to artists, former students, top digital marketers and brand designers of the world, and a few of my dear friends who are in the billion-dollar league.

Let me tell you this: I've seen so many points of view that it really made me open up my mind again. It's not what you like and what you see—it's what your customer sees. Period.

In the end, my favorite cover design was quietly voted away, and the design you're holding in your hands was (again) voted by a landslide majority. If you had asked me the same question five years ago, I wouldn't have cared at all what other people thought. I would have ultimately failed, choosing what I thought was the "perfect beautiful design."

But voilà, I tested it out—and by the time you read this book, I'm sure it'll be a bestseller because of this.

4. Don't downplay the importance of marketing. This is the key to growing yourself, your brand, and your clientele. Yes, it's expensive. But guess what else is expensive? Having to start over in a new career, especially if you've poured so much into training yourself to become a certified microblading artist. Don't make the mistake of burying yourself under a sea of other people. Invest your money where it matters: in scaling your business and allowing your skills to shine.

5. Never underestimate anyone. One negative review or nasty Instagram rant could wound your business for a long time. Better yet, treat everyone like family, because in this business, relationships are everything. It's your goal to transform every person who walks through your door into a lifelong customer. Be sure to treat your customers like gold.

6. Don't do it all by yourself. Running a business is incredibly stressful, especially when you're trying to level up in today's world. Do yourself a favor: outsource everything that you're not an expert at doing, and your stress is going to significantly decrease. With less stress, you're going to be able to run your business much more efficiently.

7. Don't use novices. While we're on the topic of outsourcing tasks, let me give you this piece of advice: delegate tasks to qualified professionals. This will save you time, effort, and money by keeping your company running efficiently. It may seem cheaper to use novices at first glance, but when you do yourself the favor of investing in trained professionals, you're putting your business on the fast track to rapid growth.

8. Never, ever stop educating yourself. I said it before, and I'll say it again: our world is changing more and more every day. It revolutionizes faster than we realize, and if you don't keep up with the changes, you're going to get left behind. Study new trends, learn new skills, and wrap your mind around new strategies to get a leg up on your competition. This isn't just the key to succeeding in business, but it's a crucial component to succeeding in life.

I believe in continuous education, reading, and always staying curious and open-minded about any idea that could help you grow. I always say that I wish I had had someone to help me through my struggles as a budding entrepreneur; someone who could have mentored me and offered support and guidance throughout the way. If I had had someone like that to help me, I would have saved myself so much time, money, and stress.

I've spent over $65,000 in the past few months solely on educating myself—learning new techniques in order to expand my knowledge of marketing, scaling, and growth—all so that I could help and support you on this journey.

If you learned a new skill, awesome, but to learn how to build a business and make real money—now that's the real deal. That's my motive here, with this book. I want to be the mentor for you that I never had. I want women of all walks of life to be able to pick up this book and realize that entrepreneurship isn't some privilege reserved for the 1% who was born wealthy—it can be achieved by anyone.

Epilogue

What's Your Dream?

In the early stages of my career, my goal was absolutely to make it into the millionaire league. And yet, as time passed and my net worth rose, my perspectives changed. After money stopped being such a big deal to me, wanted to help women achieve a beautiful look and gain confidence, and later still I wanted to teach them how to learn microblading the right way—to achieve this skill and use it to their advantage forever—but at this point in my life, my missions have changed.

Nowadays, I'm committed to helping women gain financial independence, scale their income, level up and play in a different league. Here's a secret that not many people will tell you: when you get to the top, the feeling is lonely. I want you to be a part of it—I want you to be able to fly across the globe in private jets and stay in the most exclusive resorts around the world, too. These days, *that's* my goal.

The idea of a successful business isn't just an illusion—it's achievable. And the best part? I cracked the code. I used my skills, my intuition, and my determination to understand exactly how I could make an impact in the entrepreneurial world around me. And with the lessons I've learned, I can push you forward, too.

You don't necessarily need to be a millionaire—you just need to be happy. What does "happiness" mean for you? Want to spend more time with your kids and family, all while bringing in an extra five grand a month? You can do that in a heartbeat. I already dropped so many valuable tips in this book, if you didn't grab them, then read it again. This book should be your ultimate guide on how to break free of the 9 to 5 and gain financial independence forever.

I was always pushing my students to work harder and harder, pull double-digit shifts, hustle 18 hours a day until they fell over—all so that they could get to the top of the top. But let's slow down for a second: where's the top? Get out a sheet of paper and write down your goal. And don't stop there, either; every single morning when you wake up, go to your mirror and face your biggest inspiration: yourself.

Look yourself in the eyes and repeat loudly for one minute, "I can do it." And then, say it even louder. And louder. And even louder than that. Scream it at the top of your lungs, if you have to. And when you're done, flash a smile—no, not a fake one, either. Smile your real smile; the one that paints itself across your face when you're truly, genuinely happy.

You can do it. Start each and every day with this type of attitude, and I guarantee you that you will reach the top—whatever the top means for you. But without a set goal and a proper mindset, you won't get there... because where's the goal? You don't even know where you're going if you never stop to think about it.

Personally, my goals were insane. They were realistic, but they were insane. They required me to work straight through every day (I'm talking 25-hour days), which is what I was doing until early 2018, when my 4-year-old daughter was diagnosed with autism. At that point, my entire life as I knew it shut down, and I restructured everything. My daughter was always my top priority, but making sure that she had the care she needed to develop and thrive despite her diagnosis was the number one thing on my mind—not scaling into billionaire status.

I realized that I don't need to be a billionaire to be happy and have a luxurious lifestyle. I'm a cool millionaire, and that's exactly where I want to be. This is "the top" for me: to spend time with my girl, to help her progress, and to be a luminary for women—helping you scale up around the world.

The stories of the women who joined this career path never fail to inspire me. I've witnessed their transformations firsthand, and I've seen how their lives have shifted from drab to fab. There are a variety of reasons to pursue a career in permanent makeup: either they wanted to spend more time with their kids, they wanted a little extra money, or they wanted to scale up into the big leagues of high income. Whatever the reason you get your foot in the door, this industry shapes lives and builds careers.

Earlier this year, my eyes welled up with tears when I taught a student who, like me, completely re-shifted her life when a diagnosis rocketed everything out of place. After her husband was diagnosed with Stage 4 terminal cancer, she did everything she could to provide and help him through this time. To this day, I get goosebumps when I think of this woman and the way she hustled—even at over 50 years old—courageously taking on a new career in an emerging new market, starting over later in life.

I've held the hands of 18-year-old kids who are just starting out in their careers, and I've held the hands of 65-year-old grandmothers (and some women even older than that). And what I've learned as I looked into the eyes of women from around the world, young and old, from so many different culture and backgrounds is this: it's never the wrong time to invest in yourself. It's never too early or too late to begin a new career. And most importantly, it's never the wrong time to dream a new dream.

Think of your dream…whatever that may be. I can't imagine it for you; this is where your mind runs wild. Maybe your dream is a tropical paradise, waking up in an over-water bungalow with breakfast delivered to you by canoe. Maybe your dream is to ski in the Swiss alps and spend summers in the South of France. Maybe your dream is to live in a gorgeous house with your family, never having to worry about money again. The point is that the dream is what drives you forward. The dream is what keeps you going.

It's time to ask yourself what you want out of your career. It's time to listen to the way your heels click across the floor when you walk, and feel the energy in your hands as they sculpt the confidence of women all around you. It's time to look in the mirror and see yourself for who you really are: a woman with the power in her hands to transform her life into whatever she wants it to be.

My story is unique, and so is yours. The life we all live—each and every one of us—can be hijacked and driven in any direction we please. This book should be treated as a roadmap to your success. It should be viewed as a guide on how to make the most of your time, how to maximize your years, how to create the most incredible career possible and love every second of the life you live. When you have the right mentors and coaches, you have no option other than to fly.

So let me ask you this: how high will you soar?